About the NCCN Guidelines for Patients®

National Comprehensive Cancer Network®

AF884749

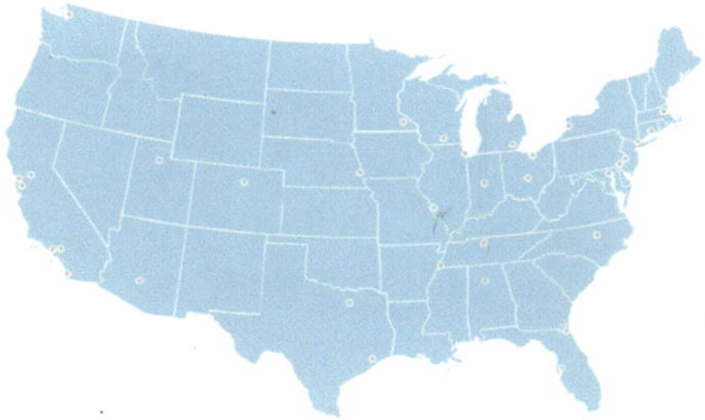

Did you know that top cancer centers across the United States work together to improve cancer care? This alliance of leading cancer centers is called the National Comprehensive Cancer Network® (NCCN®).

Cancer care is always changing. NCCN develops evidence-based cancer care recommendations used by health care providers worldwide. These frequently updated recommendations are the NCCN Clinical Practice Guidelines in Oncology (NCCN Guidelines®). The NCCN Guidelines for Patients plainly explain these expert recommendations for people with cancer and caregivers.

These NCCN Guidelines for Patients are based on the NCCN Clinical Practice Guidelines in Oncology (NCCN Guidelines®) for Adolescent and Young Adult (AYA) Oncology, Version 1.2023 – June 29, 2022.

View the NCCN Guidelines for Patients free online
NCCN.org/patientguidelines

Find an NCCN Cancer Center near you
NCCN.org/cancercenters

Connect with us YouTube

Supporters

NATIONAL COMPREHENSIVE CANCER NETWORK®
NCCN FOUNDATION
Guiding Treatment. Changing Lives.

NCCN Guidelines for Patients are supported by funding from the NCCN Foundation®

NCCN Foundation gratefully acknowledges the following corporate supporter for helping to make available these NCCN Guidelines for Patients: Servier

NCCN independently adapts, updates and hosts the NCCN Guidelines for Patients. Our corporate supporters do not participate in the development of the NCCN Guidelines for Patients and are not responsible for the content and recommendations contained therein.

Additional support is provided by

LEUKEMIA & LYMPHOMA SOCIETY®

The Leukemia & Lymphoma Society (LLS) is dedicated to developing better outcomes for blood cancer patients and their families through research, education, support and advocacy and is happy to have this comprehensive resource available to patients.
LLS.org/PatientSupport

To make a gift or learn more visit online or email

NCCNFoundation.org/donate

PatientGuidelines@NCCN.org

Contents

NCCN Foundation seeks to support the millions of patients and their families affected by a cancer diagnosis by funding and distributing NCCN Guidelines for Patients. NCCN Foundation is also committed to advancing cancer treatment by funding the nation's promising doctors at the center of innovation in cancer research. For more details and the full library of patient and caregiver resources, visit NCCN.org/patients.

National Comprehensive Cancer Network (NCCN) and NCCN Foundation
3025 Chemical Road, Suite 100, Plymouth Meeting, PA 19462 USA

1

Adolescent and young adult (AYA) cancer

An adolescent and young adult (AYA) with cancer is a person 15 to 39 years of age at the time of initial cancer diagnosis. AYAs have unique needs and challenges. Therefore, if possible, seek treatment at a cancer center with programs and services focused on the needs of AYAs with your type of cancer.

About AYAs

An adolescent and young adult (AYA) with cancer is someone 15 to 39 years of age at the time of initial cancer diagnosis. AYAs with cancer have unique medical, mental, emotional, and social concerns. This combination of mental, emotional, social, and spiritual aspects is referred to as psychosocial support. Some of the psychosocial effects of cancer are changes in how a person thinks, their feelings, moods, beliefs, ways of coping, and relationships with family, friends, and co-workers. There are different kinds of psychosocial support, including counseling, education, group support, and spiritual support

AYAs with cancer have specific age-related challenges and concerns such as:

- Fertility and fertility preservation
- Education and schooling
- Employment
- Parenting
- Childcare
- Long-term side effects or late effects
- Health insurance and living expenses
- Transportation to appointments
- Psychosocial support
- Access to services

The range of cancer types that affect AYAs is unique and different from cancers that affect younger children or older adults. Not all cancer doctors (oncologists) have experience treating AYAs. It is important that you seek out a health care provider who specializes in AYA cancer treatment.

AYAs with cancer have unique medical, mental, emotional, and social concerns.

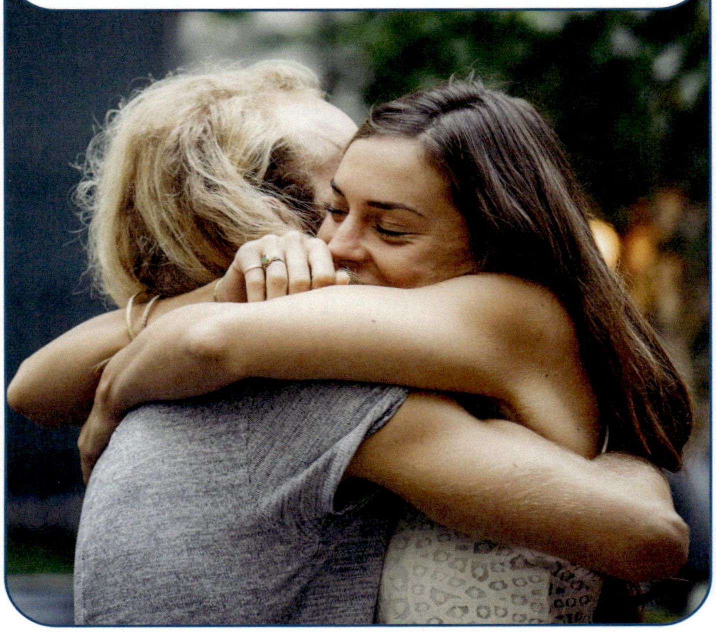

AYA cancer treatment

AYAs develop different types of cancer than other age groups. These cancers look and behave differently than the same cancers in younger children and older adults. Therefore, AYA cancer treatment is complex. AYA bodies are still going through physical and hormonal changes. These changes affect how cancer develops and how the cancer responds to treatment. Both the type of cancer you have and the age at which you were diagnosed play a role in how your cancer will be treated. And, treatment options will vary based on your unique needs.

The National Comprehensive Cancer Network® believes that the best management of anyone with cancer is in a clinical trial. NCCN encourages you to ask your health care provider if a clinical trial is available for your type of cancer. Clinical trials are more likely to be available at cancer centers that have AYA programs.

AYA cancer centers

AYAs are a unique group that can be treated by pediatric or adult oncologists in pediatric or adult centers depending on the type of cancer and the age of the person with cancer. AYA cancer centers provide a multidisciplinary and integrative approach. This includes a team of providers with expertise in AYA cancer treatment and management of specific mental health and developmental issues of AYAs.

Finding a clinical trial

In the United States

NCCN Cancer Centers
NCCN.org/cancercenters

The National Cancer Institute (NCI)
cancer.gov/about-cancer/treatment/clinical-trials/search

Worldwide

The U.S. National Library of Medicine (NLM)
clinicaltrials.gov/

Need help finding a clinical trial?

NCI's Cancer Information Service (CIS)
1.800.4.CANCER (1.800.422.6237)
cancer.gov/contact

Many cancer centers have established AYA programs to accommodate the specific needs of AYAs with cancer. AYAs are encouraged to seek care at centers with established social, clinical, therapeutic, and psychosocial support programs. We encourage you to ask your health care provider for a referral to a cancer center that has an AYA program.

Key points

- An adolescent and young adult (AYA) with cancer is someone 15 to 39 years of age at the time of initial cancer diagnosis.
- AYAs develop different types of cancer than other age groups. These cancers look and behave differently than the same cancers in younger children and older adults and are best treated by a cancer program that treats AYAs. Treatment in a clinical trial is encouraged.
- AYAs are a unique group that can be treated by pediatric or adult oncologists in pediatric or adult centers depending on the type of cancer and the age of the person with cancer.
- Many cancer centers have established AYA programs to accommodate the specific needs of AYAs with cancer. Seek out a health care provider or cancer center that specializes in AYA cancer treatment.

Seek out a health care provider, cancer center, or hospital experienced in treating AYAs with your type of cancer.

2

Fertility (all genders)

Treatment can impact fertility or the ability to have children. Therefore, it is recommended you consider fertility preservation before starting treatment. This chapter offers more information about fertility risks and steps you can take to preserve your fertility.

Understanding the risks

Some cancer treatments can harm the reproductive system and affect the ability to have children. The impact on fertility depends on the location of the cancer that will be treated, the type of treatment, and the intensity or combination of drugs. The reproductive system includes the ovaries, fallopian tubes, uterus, cervix, vagina, prostate, testes, and penis, and even specific parts of the brain.

Examples of treatments that affect the reproductive system include:

- High-dose or targeted radiation to places like the pelvic area
- A type of chemotherapy that includes alkylating agents and others that affect fertility
- Surgery to remove tissue or organs from the reproductive area

Your care team should be able to explain whether your cancer and/or cancer treatment puts your fertility at risk, and if so, how high of a risk. While it is your treatment team's responsibility to discuss this with you, it is important that you advocate for yourself and ask about fertility risk.

Discuss with your care team and a fertility specialist what can be done to:

- Limit the damage from treatment
- Protect your fertility so you have the choice to plan a pregnancy in the future
- Understand your fertility options

Some types of fertility preservation take a couple of days, and some types can take about two and half weeks. Talk to your care team about the risks of delaying treatment and any concerns you may have. Together, you and your care will decide the timing of fertility preservation.

Fertility

If you think you want children in the future, ask your care team how cancer and cancer treatment might change your fertility. In order to preserve your fertility, you may need to take action before starting cancer treatment. Those who want to have children in the future should be referred to a fertility specialist to discuss the options before starting treatment.

Changes in fertility

Treatment might cause your fertility to be interrupted or impaired. This loss can be temporary or permanent and is related to your age at time of diagnosis, treatment type(s), treatment dose, and treatment length.

- **In those assigned male at birth,** sometimes the testicles can no longer make sperm (a condition known as azoospermia) or the pathways that sperm travel through get blocked or damaged.
- **In those assigned female at birth,** sometimes the ovaries no longer release eggs, a condition called premature ovarian failure or early menopause. When there is damage to the uterus or other parts of the reproductive system, it can prevent the eggs from getting fertilized or fertilized eggs from implanting and growing inside the uterus.

Oncofertility team

The oncofertility team focuses on endocrine (hormone) health and fertility options of someone with cancer before and after treatment. Fertility preservation is all about keeping your options open, whether you know you want to have children later in life or aren't really sure at the moment. Reproductive specialists and the members of an oncofertility team can help you sort through what may work for you. Often, cancer centers that specialize in treating AYAs also have oncofertility teams or reproductive specialists.

Depending on the type of cancer and the specialists available in your area, your oncofertility team may include:

- **Your oncology care team** should start the conversation about cancer-related changes in fertility and help you understand the risks.
- **A nurse navigator or case manager** will help you navigate the referral process, coordinate the various specialists involved in your care, and deal with the insurance company.
- **An endocrinologist and fertility/reproductive specialist** can explain your fertility preservation options, including how it is done, success rates, timing, and costs. This specialist might carry out the fertility-sparing procedure.
- **A genetics counselor** can assess your risk of passing on genetic abnormalities to your children. This is usually done within the first 2 months of starting treatment.

- **A gynecologist or urologist** can assess your risk of altered fertility and guide you in addressing your fertility needs.
- **A gynecologic or urologic oncologist** specializes in cancers of the reproductive and urinary tract organs. This is usually a surgeon and may be the one to perform fertility-sparing surgery.
- **A family-planning specialist** can offer information about many different options for becoming a parent.
- **An adoption professional** can provide information and counseling on the process of becoming an adoptive parent. This can include criteria, timing, and costs.
- **A social worker or mental health provider** can give emotional support, provide financial resources, and counseling as you consider your fertility options.

Out-of-pocket costs

Often, insurance does not cover fertility preservation services. This means there are out-of-pocket costs. However, your cancer team or fertility specialists should be able to discuss the cost to fertility preservation and what discounts might be available for those with cancer.

What should I consider?

Before you decide how, or if, to preserve your fertility, think about your answer to the following questions:

- ✓ How do you feel about having children in the future?
- ✓ Have you always wanted children?
- ✓ How many children do you want to have? When?
- ✓ How do you feel about adoption?
- ✓ How would you feel about using donor sperm, eggs, or embryos?
- ✓ How would you feel about having a surrogate carry and give birth to your child?
- ✓ Do you have any religious or moral concerns about technologies such as in vitro fertilization (IVF) or embryo transplantation?

All fertility preservation methods have an out-of-pocket cost. Check with your insurance company about which fertility preservation methods are covered and what your out-of-pocket costs might be.

Preserving fertility before treatment

Your fertility preservation options will vary depending on your age, gender/sex assigned at birth, and type of cancer you have. Most techniques that can increase your chances of having children in the future must be done before starting cancer treatment. Fertility preservation involves techniques that prevent damage and remove healthy cells (sperm, eggs, or embryos) and store them for later use. Fertility preservation options can be found in **Guide 1**.

Damage prevention

Below are options used to prevent damage to the ovaries.

- **Fertility-sparing surgery** – The reproductive organs can be protected through fertility-sparing surgery. The surgeon removes only the cancerous tissue leaving as much healthy tissue in place as possible. For example, the surgeon could leave the healthy ovary in place if you have early-stage ovarian cancer. In radiation therapy, a special shield made of lead is used to prevent radiation from damaging the ovaries or testicles.
- **Ovarian transposition (oophoropexy)** – This method can prevent damage to the ovaries during radiation therapy. A surgeon will move the healthy ovary (or ovaries) out of the radiation field and attach it to the wall of your abdomen. An oophoropexy is a proven option to preserve fertility.

Banking healthy cells

Below is a list of proven and reliable methods for fertility preservation.

- **Egg freezing (oocyte cryopreservation)** – This procedure uses hormone shots, which may delay treatment, to make the ovaries produce multiple eggs. These eggs are removed and frozen, but not fertilized. This process usually takes about two and half weeks.
- **Embryo freezing (embryo cryopreservation) after in vitro fertilization (IVF)** – In this process, eggs are removed from the ovaries and fertilized with sperm in a lab. The embryo is then frozen. IVF can be done using a sperm donor. IVF involves a series of hormone shots to prompt the ovaries to produce more than one egg. This process usually takes about two and half weeks.
- **Ovarian tissue freezing (cryopreservation)** – The surgical removal and freezing of a healthy ovary (or part of an ovary). After cancer treatment, the tissue is put back into the body.
- **Sperm banking (sperm cryopreservation)** – This procedure collects and freezes one or more samples of ejaculate (semen). Sperm banking kits can be ordered online or you can make an appointment at a local urology office.
- **Testicular sperm extraction** – This is the removal of a sperm from the testicle while under local anesthesia (a controlled loss of feeling in a small area of the body from drugs). Sperm cells are then frozen.

Other options

The option below might not be available or appropriate for you.

- **Testicular tissue freezing (cryopreservation)** – The surgical removal of a small portion of tissue from the testicle. The tissue is frozen to make sperm from it later.

Guide 1
Fertility preservation options

Egg freezing (oocyte cryopreservation)	A process in which eggs are removed from the ovaries and frozen.
Embryo freezing (embryo cryopreservation) after in vitro fertilization (IVF)	A process in which eggs are removed from the ovaries and fertilized by sperm in a lab to create an embryo. The embryo is frozen.
Ovarian transposition (oophoropexy)	A surgeon will move the healthy ovary (or ovaries) out of the radiation field and attach it to the wall of your abdomen.
Ovarian tissue freezing (cyropreservation)	A surgeon removes the ovary or part of it and freezes it. After cancer treatment, the ovary or tissue is put back. This option is not always available.
Sperm banking (sperm cryopreservation)	A procedure that collects and freezes one or more samples of semen. Sperm banking kits can be ordered online or you can make an appointment at a local urology office.
Testicular sperm extraction	A surgeon removes sperm cells directly from the testicle. The sperm cells are frozen.
Testicular tissue freezing (cryopreservation)	A surgeon removes a small portion of tissue from the testicle and freezes it to try to make sperm from it later. This option is not always available.

Fertility after treatment

A follow-up with a fertility specialist after treatment may be helpful. If you noticed changes in your fertility, then consider the following possible options:

- **Donor eggs or embryos** – Donor eggs are removed from someone other than you. The donor goes through hormone treatment to produce multiple eggs. Donor eggs are fertilized through IVF using sperm chosen by you. Some people donate their frozen embryos for someone else to use.
- **Adoption or fostering** – Some adoption agencies may require that you be cancer-free (in remission) and off treatment for a certain amount of time before adopting a child. You could also become a foster parent. For more information, consider state, national, and federal organizations like ChildWelfare.gov or AdoptUsKids.org.
- **Surrogate pregnancy** – In a surrogate pregnancy, a frozen embryo is created from the egg and sperm from you and a designated partner. The embryo is implanted in the uterus of a surrogate chosen by you, who carries the baby until birth. Often, there is a legal agreement between the person who will become pregnant and the future parent(s).

Those who want to have children in the future should be referred to a fertility specialist to discuss the options before starting treatment.

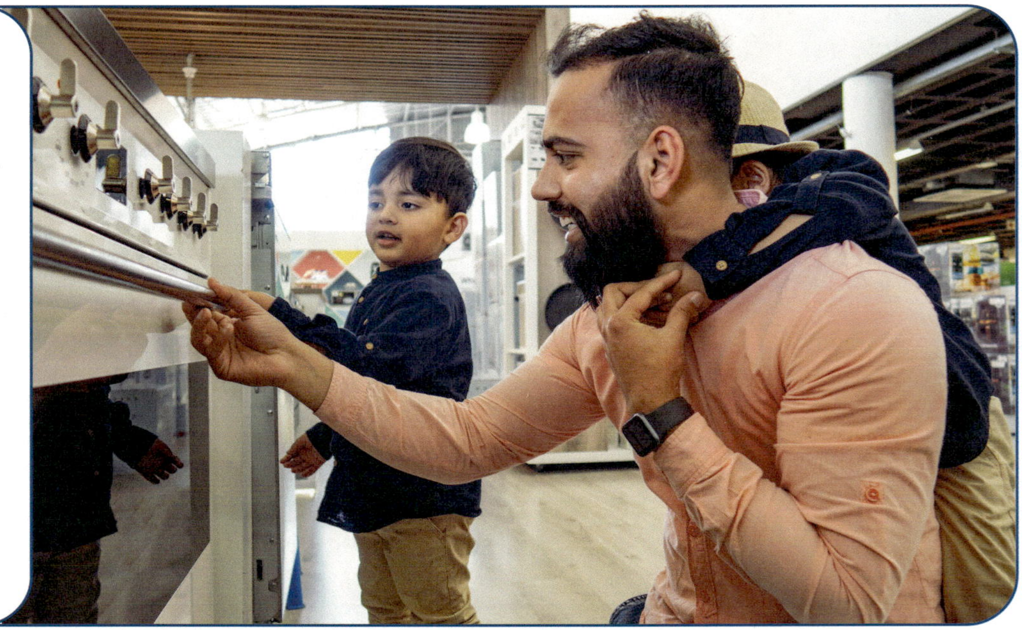

Preventing pregnancy during treatment

Avoiding pregnancy during cancer therapy is very important. Becoming pregnant, or having your partner becoming pregnant during chemotherapy, radiation therapy, or other types of systemic therapy may lead to serious birth defects. Because, cancer and cancer treatment can affect the ovaries and damage sperm.

Hormonal birth control may or may not be recommended, so ask your care team about intrauterine devices (IUDs), condoms, diaphragms, cervical caps, and the contraceptive sponge.

Speak to your care team about preventing pregnancy while being treated for cancer. Those who want to become pregnant in the future should be referred to a fertility specialist to discuss the options before starting treatment.

Those with ovaries

Those who can become pregnant will have a pregnancy test before starting treatment. Cancer treatment can hurt the developing baby if you are or become pregnant during treatment. Therefore, birth control to prevent pregnancy during and after treatment is recommended. If you are pregnant or breastfeeding at the time of your cancer diagnosis, certain treatments will need to be avoided.

Menstruation, menses, menstrual flow, or your "period" may stop during treatment, but often returns within 2 years after treatment in those 40 years of age and under. It is still possible to become pregnant even though you might not have a period. Therefore, birth control is recommended during and after treatment. Consult your care team for the best time to plan a pregnancy.

Blood clots

Venous thromboembolism (VTE) refers to blood clots in the veins. If you are at risk of VTE, your care team will recommend specific contraceptive methods.

Those with testicles

Cancer and cancer treatment can damage sperm. Sperm counts can return a few years after treatment is completed. Use contraception (birth control) such as condoms to prevent pregnancy during and immediately after cancer treatment.

Key points

- Ask your care team how cancer and cancer treatment will change your fertility and sexual health now and in the future. Know the risks.
- Seek a referral for a fertility preservation specialist if treatment might impact your fertility and you want to take steps to protect your fertility. A medical professional, social worker, or counselor can help you decide on what is best for you.
- Your fertility preservation options will vary depending on your age, gender/sex assigned at birth, and type of cancer you have. If you think you might want children in the future, talk to your doctor now.
- Sperm banking and testicular sperm extraction are reliable and proven methods of fertility preservation.
- Embryo freezing, egg freezing, and ovarian transposition are reliable and proven methods of fertility preservation.
- Preventing pregnancy during treatment is important. Hormonal birth control may or may not be recommended, so ask your care team about options.

share with us.

Take our survey.
And help make the
NCCN Guidelines for Patients
better for everyone!

NCCN.org/patients/comments

3

Testing and treatment

Not all cancers are the same. Accurate testing is needed to diagnose and treat cancer. Treatment planning starts with testing. Together, you and your care team will choose a treatment plan that is right for you.

Test results

Accurate testing is needed to diagnose and treat cancer. Results from imaging studies and biopsies will be used to determine your treatment plan. It is important you understand what these tests mean. Ask questions and keep copies of your test results. Online patient portals are a great way to access your test results.

Keep these things in mind:

- Choose a friend, family member, or peer who can drive you to appointments, provide meals, or offer emotional support during diagnosis and treatment.
- Bring someone with you to doctor visits, if possible.
- Write down questions and take notes during appointments. Don't be afraid to ask your care team questions. Get to know your care team and help them get to know you.
- Get copies of blood tests, imaging results, and reports about the specific type of cancer you have.
- Organize your papers. Create files for insurance forms, medical records, and test results. You can do the same on your computer.
- Keep a list of contact information for everyone on your care team. Add it to your phone. Hang the list on your refrigerator or keep it in a place where someone can access it in an emergency. Keep your primary care physician (PCP) informed of changes to this list. You are encouraged to keep your PCP. They are great partners in care.
- Include in your contact list information on the exact subtype of cancer, as well as any treatment and the date it started.

Testing takes time. It might take days or weeks for all test results to come in.

Genetic and genetic risk testing

You might be thinking why did I get cancer? Most of the time, the answer is one cell made a mistake when dividing and then a cancer formed. Some, however, have a predisposition or have something in their DNA (genetic material) that makes them more likely to develop cancer. AYAs are more likely to have a cancer predisposition condition than older adults with cancer. Understanding whether you have a cancer predisposition condition can sometimes affect your cancer treatment, but more often, it can affect screening for other cancers. Therefore, identifying a cancer predisposition condition is important.

Genetic testing is done using blood or saliva (spitting into a cup). The goal is to look for gene mutations inherited from your biological parents called germline mutations. Some mutations can put you at risk for more than one type of cancer. You can pass these genes on to your children. Also, family members might carry these mutations. Tell your care team if there is a family history of cancer.

A genetic risk assessment will identify if you carry a cancer risk and if you may benefit from genetic testing, additional screening, or preventive interventions. Depending on the genetic risk assessment, you might undergo genetic testing and genetic counseling.

Create a medical binder

A medical binder or notebook is a great way to organize all of your records in one place.

- ✓ Make copies of blood tests, imaging results, and reports about your specific type of cancer. It will be helpful when getting a second opinion.
- ✓ Choose a binder that meets your needs. Consider a zipper pocket to include a pen, small calendar, and insurance cards.
- ✓ Create folders for insurance forms, test types (blood, imaging, pathology, radiology, genetics), treatments, and procedures. Organize items in the folder by date.
- ✓ Use online patient portals to view your test results and other records. Download or print the records to add to your binder.
- ✓ Add a section for questions and to take notes.

Bring your medical binder to appointments. You never know when you might need it!

Biomarker testing

Inside our cells are deoxyribonucleic acid (DNA) molecules. These molecules are tightly packaged into what is called a chromosome. Chromosomes contain most of the genetic information in a cell. Normal human cells contain 23 pairs of chromosomes for a total of 46 chromosomes. Each chromosome contains thousands of genes. Genes are coded instructions for the proteins your cells make. A mutation is when something goes wrong in the genetic code.

A sample from your biopsy will undergo lab tests to look for specific DNA mutations/alterations, protein levels, or other molecular features. This information is used to learn more about your type of cancer and to choose the best treatment for you. It is sometimes called molecular testing, tumor profiling, gene expression profiling, or genomic testing.

Biomarker testing includes tests of genes or their products (proteins). It identifies the presence or absence of mutations and certain proteins that might suggest treatment. Proteins are written like this: BRCA. Genes are written with italics like this: *BRCA*. When a gene or protein is found, it shown with a plus sign (+) like this: CD10+. When it has not been found, it will be written with a negative sign (-) like this CD10-.

What is your family health history?

Some cancers and other diseases run in families – those who are related to you through genes passed down from parent to child. This information is called a family health history. You can ask family members about their health issues like heart disease, cancer, and diabetes, and at what age they were diagnosed. For relatives who have died, ask about the cause and age of death.

Start by asking your parents, siblings, and children. Next, talk to half-siblings, aunts and uncles, nieces and nephews, grandparents, and grandchildren.

Write down what you learn about your family history and share with your health care provider.

Some of the questions to ask include:

- Do you have any chronic diseases, such as heart disease or diabetes, or health conditions such as high blood pressure or high cholesterol?
- Have you had any other diseases, such as cancer or stroke?
- How old were you when each of these diseases and health conditions was diagnosed?
- What is our family's ancestry – from what countries did our ancestors originate?

Care team

Treating cancer takes a team approach. Treatment decisions should involve a multidisciplinary team (MDT). An MDT is a team of doctors, nurses, health care providers, and psychosocial professionals from different professional backgrounds who have knowledge (expertise) and experience in AYAs with your type of cancer. This team is united in the planning and implementing of your treatment. Ask who will coordinate your care.

Some members of your care team will be with you throughout cancer treatment, while others will only be there for parts of it. Get to know your care team and help them get to know you. It is important to have regular talks with your care team about your goals for treatment and your treatment plan.

Depending on your diagnosis, your team might include the following:

- **A diagnostic radiologist** interprets the results of x-rays and other imaging tests.
- **An interventional radiologist** performs needle biopsies and places ports for treatment.
- **A medical oncologist** treats cancer in adults using systemic therapy.
- **A radiation oncologist** prescribes and plans radiation therapy to treat cancer.
- **A hematologist or hematologic oncologist** is a medical expert in blood diseases and blood cancers.
- **A pathologist or hematopathologist** analyzes the cells and tissues removed during a biopsy and provides cancer diagnosis, staging, and information about biomarker testing.
- **An anesthesiologist** gives anesthesia, a medicine so you do not feel pain during surgery or procedures.
- **Residents and fellows** are doctors who are continuing their training, some to become specialists in a certain field of medicine.
- **Nurse practitioners (NPs) and physician assistants (PAs)** are health care providers. Some of your clinic visits may be done by a nurse practitioner or physician assistant.
- **Oncology nurses** provide your hands-on care, like giving systemic therapy, managing your care, answering questions, and helping you cope with side effects.
- **Oncology pharmacists** provide medicines used to treat cancer and to manage symptoms and side effects.
- **Palliative care nurses, advanced practice providers (APPs), and physicians** help provide cancer care, may prescribe necessary medicines, and provide an extra layer of support with your cancer-related symptoms.
- **Nutritionists and dietitians** can provide guidance on what foods are most suitable for your condition.
- **An occupational therapist** helps people with the tasks of daily living.
- **A physical therapist** helps people move with greater comfort and ease.
- **A certified lymphedema therapist** gives a type of massage called manual lymph drainage.

- **Psychologists and psychiatrists** are mental health experts who can help treat and manage issues such as depression, anxiety, or other mental health conditions that can affect how you think and feel.
- **Social workers** help people solve and cope with problems in their everyday lives. Clinical social workers also diagnose and treat mental, behavioral, and emotional issues. The anxiety and adjustment an individual and family feels when diagnosed with cancer might be managed by a social worker in some cancer centers. They, or other designated professionals, can also help navigate the complexities of financial and insurance stresses.
- **Research team** helps to collect research data and coordinate care if you are in a clinical trial.

Your physical, mental, and emotional well-being are important. You know yourself better than anyone. Help other team members understand:

- How you feel
- What you need
- What is working and what is not

Keep a list of names and contact information for each member of your care team. This will make it easier for you and anyone involved in your care to know who to contact with questions or concerns.

Get to know your care team and help them get to know you.

Treatment plan

Goals of a cancer treatment plan include:

- To cure the cancer: to get rid of all the cancer cells in your body
- To control the cancer: to keep cancer from spreading, slow its growth, or destroy cancer cells that have spread to other parts of your body
- To ease cancer symptoms (sometimes called palliation): to shrink cancer tumors that are causing pain or pressure

Treatment can affect fertility. Those who want to have children in the future should be referred to a fertility specialist before starting chemotherapy and/or radiation therapy to discuss the options.

Follow your plan

Sticking with your treatment plan is very important. Many AYAs can stray from their treatment plan at one time or another—whether it's forgetting to take medicine, missing a treatment appointment, or participating in activities or taking supplements that can cause treatment not to work as well as it could. Talk to your care team about any and all of your concerns, whether they are financial, work- or school-related, or finding childcare so you can go to doctor appointments. They are there to help!

For AYAs, and parents and caregivers of teens

- ✓ Take care of yourself. This is a stressful time. Make an appointment to see your doctor. Seek out and ask for support. Support can be a friend, relative, neighbor, or co-worker.
- ✓ This will be a confusing time. You will hear a lot of unfamiliar words. Start conversations with questions and about your concerns.
- ✓ Encourage your teen to interact with their health care team, to ask questions, and to talk about how they feel.
- ✓ Teach your teen how and when to take their medicine, what to do if their medicine is low, how to refill a prescription, how to manage side effects, and who to call if they have questions about their medicine or treatment.
- ✓ Explain to your teen why taking medicine is important. Create a chart so they can keep track of when to take medicine or use an electronic device to schedule a reminder.
- ✓ Treating AYAs with cancer is complex. Not everyone responds to treatment the same way. Some do better than expected. Others do worse. A treatment response takes time.
- ✓ Celebrate treatment milestones and other events. Find ways to engage your teen Explore new interests together.

What you can do

Pick a treatment plan that works for you. Talk to your care team about any concerns or challenges that you have. Take all of your medicine as prescribed. Take the recommended amounts, at the right time. Skipping or delaying doses may change the drug's effects. If you're having difficulty paying for medicine, ask your treatment team for help.

Supportive care

Supportive care is health care given during all cancer stages. It aims to prevent, reduce, and relieve suffering, and to improve quality of life. Supportive care might include palliative care, pain relief, emotional or spiritual support, financial aid, or family counseling. Tell your care team how you are feeling and about any side effects so they can be managed. Supportive care and palliative care are often used interchangeably.

It is very important to take care of yourself by eating well, drinking plenty of fluids, exercising, and doing things that make you feel energized. Strength is needed to sustain you during treatment.

Distress

Depression, anxiety, and sleep issues are common during and after cancer treatment. Talk to your care team and with those whom you feel most comfortable about how you are feeling. There are services, people, and medicine that can help you. Support and counseling services are available.

More information on distress can be found at NCCN.org/PatientGuidelines and on the NCCN Patient Guides for Cancer app.

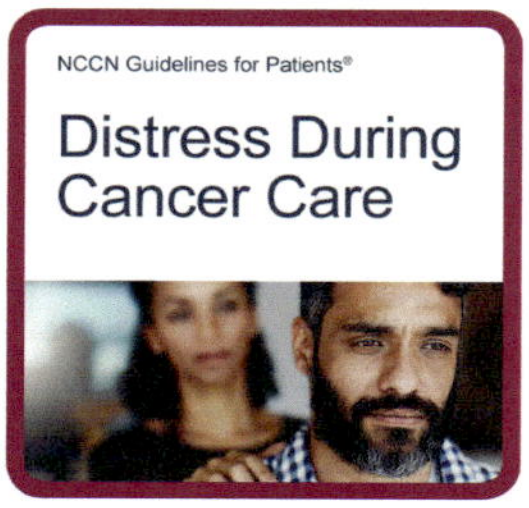

Fatigue

Fatigue is extreme tiredness and inability to function due to lack of energy. Fatigue may be caused by cancer or it may be a side effect of treatment. Let your care team know how you are feeling and if fatigue is getting in the way of doing the things you enjoy. Eating a balanced diet, exercise, yoga, and massage therapy can help. You might be referred to a nutritionist or dietitian to help with fatigue.

Financial stress

If you struggle to pay for food, housing, treatment, follow-up care, and other expenses or have difficulty getting to appointments, talk with your care team's social worker, patient navigators, and hospital financial services. They can help you find financial support and transportation options.

Late effects

Late effects are side effects that occur months or years after a disease is diagnosed or after treatment has ended. Late effects may be caused by cancer or cancer treatment. They may include changes in physical, mental, and social health, and secondary cancers. The sooner late effects are treated the better. Ask your care team about what late effects could occur. This will help you know what to expect. After your cancer treatment ends, continue follow-up visits to monitor for late effects and any risk of disease recurrence.

Lymphedema

Lymphedema is a condition in which extra lymph fluid builds up in tissues and causes swelling. It may be caused when part of the lymph system is damaged or blocked, such as during surgery to remove lymph nodes, or radiation therapy. Cancers that block lymph vessels can also cause lymphedema. Swelling usually develops slowly over time. It may develop during treatment or it may start years after treatment. If you have lymphedema, you may be referred to an expert in lymphedema management. The swelling may be reduced by exercise, massage, compression sleeves, and other means. Ask your care team about the ways to treat lymphedema.

Neurocognitive effects

Some treatments can damage the nervous system (neurotoxicity) causing problems with concentration and memory. Survivors are at risk for neurotoxicity and might be recommended for neuropsychological testing. Neuropsychology looks at how the health of your brain affects your thinking and behavior. Neuropsychological testing can identify your limits and doctors can create a plan to help with these limits.

> "After going through cancer at the age of 15, I knew that nothing in my life would ever be the same. I decided that from then on out I would live my life with gusto; I would take risks and never take anything for granted again."

Neuropathy

Neuropathy is a nerve problem that causes pain, numbness, tingling, swelling, or muscle weakness in different parts of the body. It usually begins in the hands or feet and gets worse over time. Neuropathy may be caused by cancer or cancer treatment such as chemotherapy. Ask your care team what can be done to prevent or manage neuropathy.

Pain

Tell your care team about any pain or discomfort. You might meet with a palliative care specialist or with a pain specialist to manage pain.

Key points

- Online patient portals are a great way to access your test results. Be sure to discuss these results with your care team before drawing any conclusions about what the results might mean.
- Genetic testing is done using blood or saliva (spitting into a cup). The goal is to look for gene mutations inherited from your biological parents called germline mutations.
- Biomarker testing includes tests of genes or their products (proteins). It identifies the presence or absence of mutations and certain proteins that might suggest treatment.
- A multidisciplinary team (MDT) is a team of doctors, nurses, health care providers, and psychosocial care professionals from different professional backgrounds who have knowledge (expertise) and experience in AYAs with your type of cancer.
- A treatment plan is a written course of action that covers every stage of the treatment process. Most AYAs with cancer go through several rounds of treatment. Pick a treatment plan you can follow.
- Treatment can affect fertility in all genders. Those who want to have children in the future should be referred to a fertility specialist before starting treatment to discuss the options.
- Supportive care is health care that relieves symptoms caused by cancer or its treatment and improves quality of life. Supportive care should be included in every stage of cancer treatment and be part of your treatment plan.
- All cancer treatments can cause unwanted health issues called side effects. It is important for you to tell your care team about all your side effects so they can be managed.
- Eating a balanced diet, drinking enough fluids, exercise, yoga, and massage therapy can help manage side effects.
- Some side effects, called late effects, may take years to appear. Risk for late effects will depend on the type(s) of cancer treatment you had, and the dose and the length of time you were treated. It is important to keep follow-up appointments.

Need help paying for medicine or treatment?

Ask your care team what options are available.

4

Life after treatment

An individual is considered a cancer survivor from the time of diagnosis and throughout life. After treatment, you will be monitored for any new or ongoing health issues. It is important to keep any follow-up doctor visits and imaging test appointments.

Some of the most important things you can do for your health after treatment are basic, but that doesn't mean they are easy! These things include getting enough sleep, getting quality sleep, eating a healthful diet containing mostly plant-based and non-processed foods, and incorporating a daily movement or exercise routine. Additional healthful things to consider include maintaining a strong social connection to others, limiting alcohol, and not smoking or vaping.

Follow-up care

Long-term follow-up care is very important to a cancer survivor. Even though treatment is over, you will still need to see your health care providers who will monitor for treatment-related side effects, the return of cancer, and other health changes. Seek good routine medical care, including regular doctor visits for preventive care and cancer screening. Cancer-specific tests and screenings may be recommended. It is important to keep any follow-up doctor visits and imaging test appointments.

It is your cancer treatment team's responsibility to provide you with information about your long-term risks including a survivorship care plan. Ideally, you will be followed in a cancer survivorship clinic. Ask your team about a referral.

Late effects

Some survivors have few or no health issues. Many have ongoing health challenges caused by cancer treatment and surgery. Some symptoms take time to show up, called late effects. Your risk for late effects will depend on the type(s) of cancer treatment you had, and the dose and the length of time you were treated. AYA cancer survivors have a high risk of developing a wide range of late effects. It is important to go to your follow-up appointments. The sooner late effects are treated the better. Ask your care team about what late effects could occur. This will help you know what to look for.

Possible late effects from cancer treatment:

- Secondary cancers
- Heart, lung, and kidney concerns
- Hearing and vision changes
- Fertility changes

General health

All cancer survivors are monitored for long-term side effects. Side effects can be managed. Talk to your health care provider (HCP) about how you are feeling.

In general:

- Maintain your weight.
- Adopt a physically active lifestyle. The goal is at least 30 minutes of moderate intensity activity most days of the week.
- Eat a mostly plant-based diet.
- Limit alcohol.
- Avoid tobacco products. If you smoke or vape, seek help to quit.

Blood disorders

You might be at higher risk for blood disorders such as acute myeloid leukemia (AML) or myelodysplasia (MDS) if you were exposed to heavy metals, some types of systemic (drug) therapy, or had a hematopoietic (stem) cell transplant (HCT).

More information on AML and MDS can be found at NCCN.org/patientguidelines and on the NCCN Patient Guides for Cancer app.

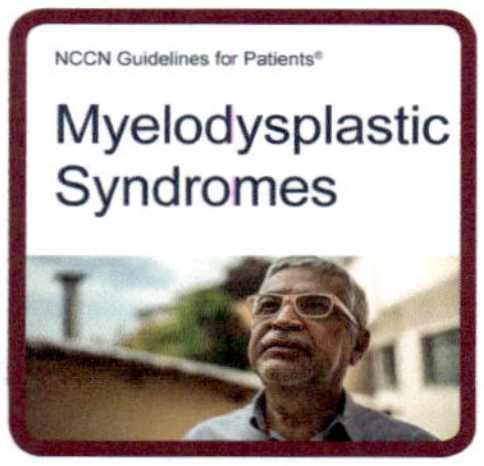

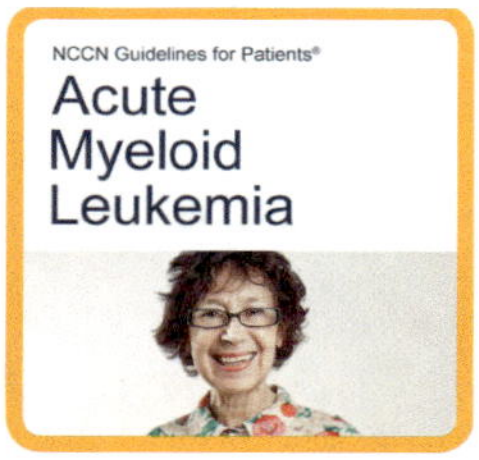

Graft-versus-host disease

If you had a donor stem cell transplant called an allogeneic hematopoietic cell transplant (alloHCT), then you will be monitored for graft-versus-host disease (GVHD). In GVHD, the donor cells attack your normal, healthy tissue. There are treatments for GVHD.

More information on GVHD can be found at NCCN.org/patientguidelines and on the NCCN Patient Guides for Cancer app.

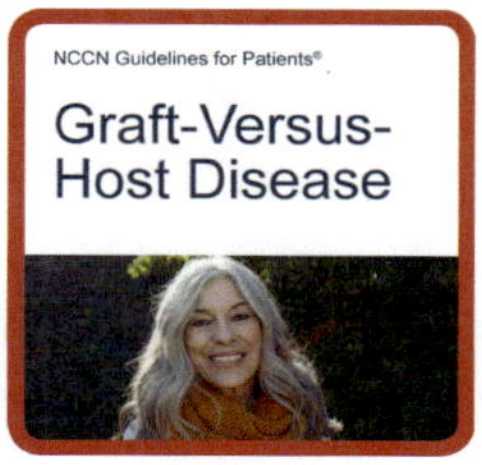

Hearing

Some treatments can affect hearing. Hearing (audiology) testing might be recommended.

Heart

Certain treatments can affect heart (cardiac) function. Heart tests might be recommended to see how well your heart works. You might be referred to a cardiologist or an onco-cardiologist. Everyone should have their blood pressure and cholesterol levels monitored on a yearly basis.

Kidneys and bladder

The kidneys filter blood to remove waste, extra water, and substances such as those used in cancer treatment. The bladder holds this waste in the form of urine before it leaves the body. Cancer drugs can collect in and harm the kidneys and bladder. Blood tests and blood pressure readings can help monitor the health of your kidneys. Let your heath care provider know if you have bladder pain, difficulty urinating, or are prone to urinary tract infections.

Lungs and breathing

Lung and breathing (pulmonary) issues such as asthma, chronic cough, emphysema, lung fibrosis, recurrent pneumonia, and shortness of breath can occur in AYA survivors. Therefore, avoid tobacco products. If you vape or smoke, seek help to quit. If you were treated with radiation therapy and certain types of systemic therapy, then you might undergo lung function screening.

Neuroendocrine

Neuroendocrine is the interaction between the nervous system and endocrine system. It describes certain cells that release hormones into the blood in response to stimulation of the nervous system. Radiation to certain areas of the body can affect hormone levels. Ask your health care provider (HCP) what screening might be recommended.

Neurocognitive or neuropsychological effects

Some treatments can damage the nervous system (neurotoxicity) causing problems with concentration, memory, and thinking. Survivors are at risk for neurotoxicity and might be recommended for neuropsychological testing. Neuropsychology looks at how the health of your brain affects your thinking and behavior. Neuropsychological testing can identify your limits and a health care professional can create a plan to help with these limits.

Skin

Those who had radiation therapy as part of a treatment plan are at risk for developing skin lesions, cancer, or other skin-related conditions. However, a yearly skin exam performed by a dermatologist is recommended for everyone.

"As AYAs, we're not relying on our parents anymore. We might not have our own insurance. Ask for help. Ask for resources. There are many people who want to support you."

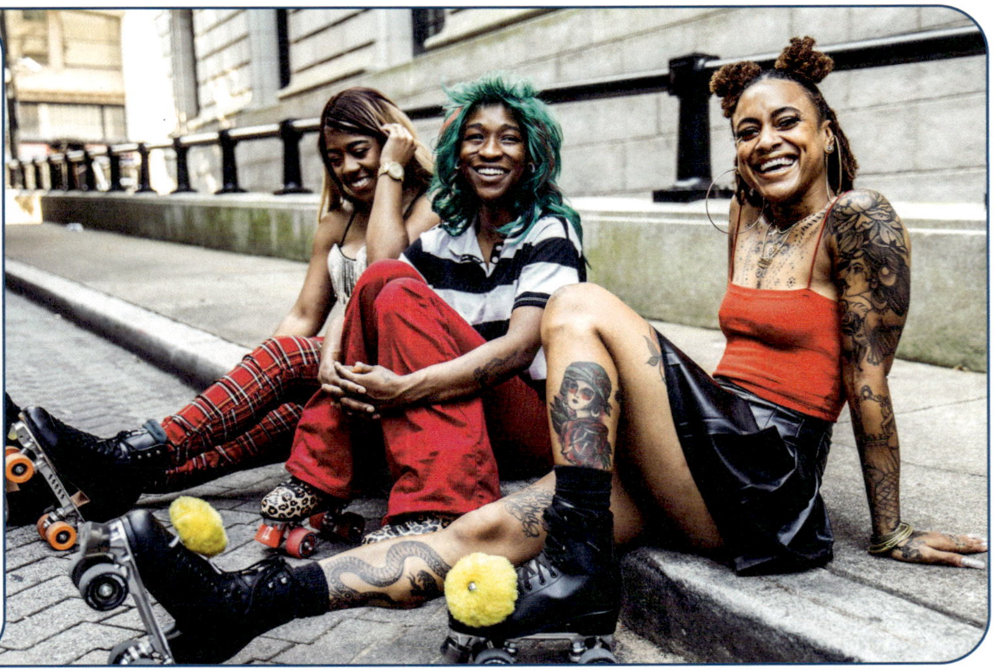

Thyroid

Prior radiation to the thyroid gland can increase the risk for thyroid disorders such as hypothyroidism (very common), thyroid cancer (common), and hyperthyroidism (uncommon). Thyroid screening may be recommended.

Cancer screenings

Schedule cancer screenings and vaccinations as recommended by your HCP based on your age, risk, and other factors.

Screenings for cancer include:

- Breast
- Colorectal
- Esophagus
- Lung
- Prostate
- Skin

Vaccinations

Vaccinations and immunizations aim to prevent or reduce the likelihood of infection, serious illness, and death caused by a specific virus or bacteria. Vaccination is the use of a vaccine to give you immunity to a disease. Vaccines cause an immune response that helps the body recognize and destroy bacteria, viruses, or cancer cells. Immunization is the process by which you become protected against a disease. Depending on the time since you completed cancer treatment and the type of cancer you had, your HCP might need to consult a specialist to understand the best timing for certain vaccinations.

AYA cancer survivors should receive the following recommend vaccinations:

- HPV vaccine for all survivors aged 9 to 26 years
- COVID-19 vaccination and boosters, see the NCCN COVID-19 Vaccination Guide for People with Cancer at NCCN.org/covid-19

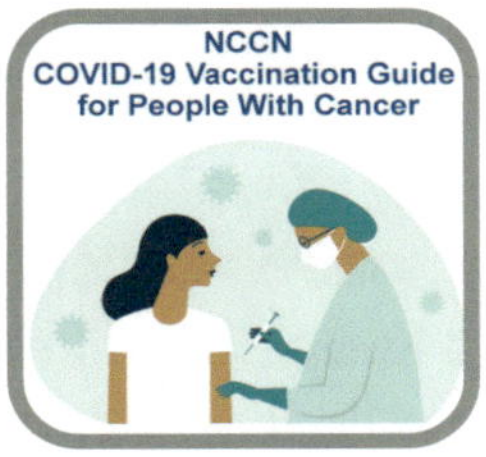

- Annual influenza (flu) vaccine
- Other vaccinations or re-vaccination may be recommended based on your age and overall health

Keep follow-up visits and imaging test appointments. Seek good routine medical care, including preventive care and cancer screenings.

Secondary cancers

AYA survivors may be at risk for developing another cancer or secondary cancer. This is not the return or recurrence of your original cancer, but a different cancer as a result of treatment with radiation and/or systemic (drug) therapy. The type of secondary cancer depends on the age when you were diagnosed with the original cancer, type and dose of systemic, and/or location and dose of radiation therapy. It is important to take care of yourself by eating well, drinking plenty of water, avoiding tobacco products and recreational drugs, limiting alcohol, and keeping wellness visits, health screenings, medical and dental appointments, and follow-up blood and imaging testing.

AYAs, especially those with risk factors, should be made aware of the importance of early diagnosis and self-examination of the skin, breasts, and testicles as recommended by the American Cancer Society. Ask your HCP for more information and your risk for developing certain cancers. Risk for developing cancer may or may not be related to your disease, treatment, family history, or other health issues. Certain cancer screenings are recommended for everyone.

Colorectal cancer

Screening for colorectal cancers may be recommended in AYAs with inherited or family risk factors. More information on colorectal screening can be found at NCCN.org/patientguidelines and on the NCCN Patient Guides for Cancer app.

Breast cancer screening

Screening for breast cancer may be recommended in AYAs with inherited or family risk factors. More information on breast screening and diagnosis can be found at NCCN.org/patientguidelines and on the NCCN Patient Guides for Cancer app.

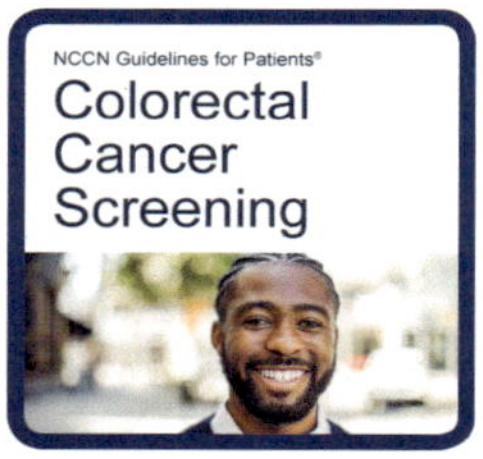

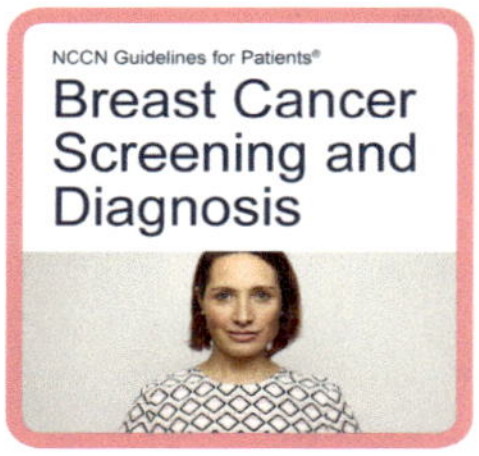

Li-Fraumeni syndrome

AYAs with Li-Fraumeni syndrome or LFS (resulting from germline mutations in the TP53 tumor suppressor gene) or germline mutations in the retinoblastoma (RB) gene are at higher risk of developing osteosarcoma and rhabdomyosarcoma.

AYAs with a family history of Li-Fraumeni syndrome have a higher risk of developing not only sarcomas but a wide variety of cancers including leukemia, brain tumors, breast cancer, and adrenocortical carcinoma before 40 years of age. Screening may be recommended by genetic counseling.

Multiple neuroendocrine neoplasia syndromes

Those with multiple neuroendocrine neoplasia (MEN) syndromes (MEN1 and MEN2) are at risk of developing multiple endocrine tumors. More information on adrenal tumors and neuroendocrine tumors can be found at NCCN.org/patientguidelines and on the NCCN Patient Guides for Cancer app.

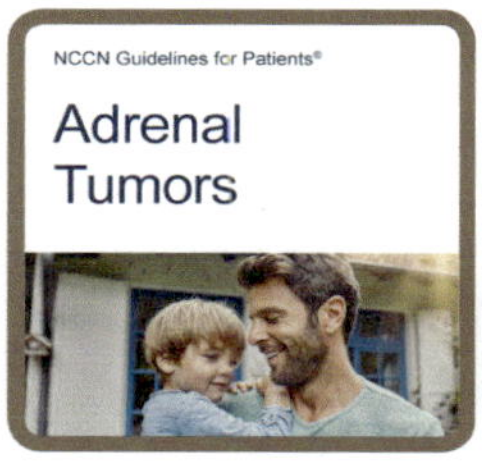

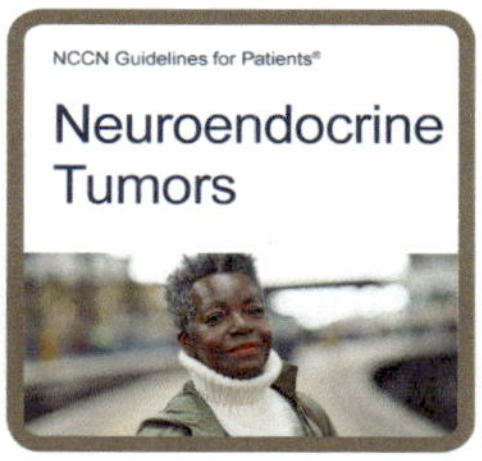

HPV

Human papillomavirus (HPV) can cause abnormal tissue growth and other changes to cells. Long-term infections with certain types of HPV can cause cervical cancer. HPV may also increase the risk of developing other types of cancer, such as anal, vaginal, vulvar, penile, and oropharyngeal cancers. HPV vaccination is recommended in adolescents 9 to 12 years of age. However, HPV vaccination can be given through 26 years of age.

More information on HPV-positive cancers can be found at NCCN.org/patientguidelines and on the NCCN Patient Guides for Cancer app.

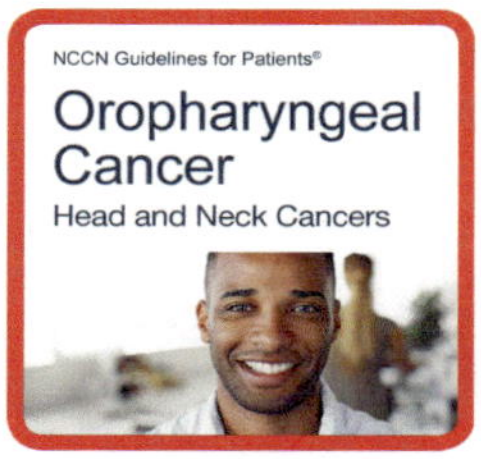

"Six months after beginning chemotherapy, I was ushered to go back to work. Despite a half-year hiatus, I felt unready to deal with the real world. My mental health tremendously declined after completing treatment; you always hear about how things will be better once you complete them, but nothing can prepare you for the changes and uncertainty you face once treatment is over."

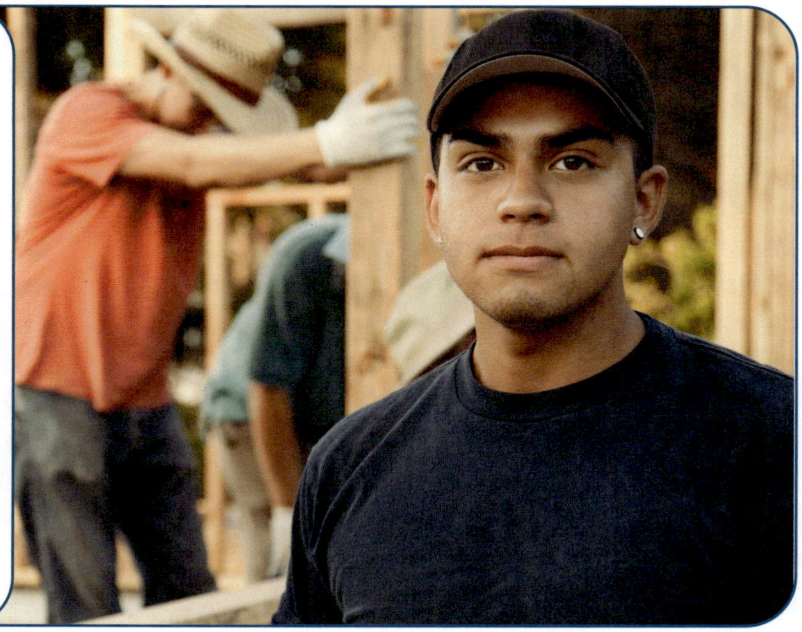

Living with and beyond cancer

Most of us probably think of a survivor as someone who has been cured of cancer. However, a person is considered a cancer survivor from the time of diagnosis and throughout life. And so, defining survivorship can be a challenge not only for the person who has or had cancer, but also a challenge for their family, friends, caregivers, or coworkers. Some people don't like the word "survivor" because it doesn't accurately describe how they feel. If you don't like the word "survivor," then choose another word. Define for yourself what it means to be someone who is living with or beyond cancer. Share with others the words you choose to represent how you feel.

Survivorship focuses on the physical, social, emotional, and financial issues unique to cancer survivors. Managing the long-term side effects of cancer and its treatment, staying connected with your primary care doctor, and living a healthy lifestyle are important parts of survivorship. Cancer survivors may experience both short- and long-term health effects of cancer and its treatment. These effects are different for everyone and depend on the treatment(s) received.

Milestones

Many cancer survivors have mixed emotions about milestones and anniversaries of certain cancer-related dates. Not everyone wants to celebrate the end of treatment or the anniversary of being cancer-free. Your feelings might change over time or from year-to-year. Prepare yourself in advance for anniversary dates, consider ways to sort through complex emotions, and decide if you want to reflect on your experiences.

Support from others

Family, friends, and coworkers can find it difficult to know how and when to support a person who has or had cancer. Reach out to others when you need help. Healing and recovery from the experience will take time. Everyone is different. Be clear whether or not you want to celebrate a milestone or anniversary. It's okay to change your mind!

Distress

Distress, depression, and anxiety are common among AYA cancer survivors. Counseling and practical support will help you during and after cancer treatment. Seek out peer support groups. Talk to your care team. Ask for a referral to a specialist or other professional who can help.

Stress and coping

Coping skills are strategies a person uses to deal with stressful situations. These skills can be learned and each person has a different way of coping. Eating a balanced diet, exercise, quality sleep, and fun or relaxing activities can help. Reach out for support to manage stress and build coping strategies.

Life changes

Being a cancer survivor can add new layers of complexity to your personal life and relationships. You may question who to tell about your history, how much they need to know, and when you should tell them. It can take time to recover from the effects of cancer treatment. Survivors may take on too much. Friends and family may not realize you still need their support.

Surviving cancer can also give you a new point of view on life and what you want from it. You may find new ways to take advantage of what life brings your way or set new goals for your future.

At school

Challenges with concentration and memory can make it hard to get back to your school life. Try cutting back on your course load. Plan more time to study and to complete assignments. If any treatment-related side effects are making it hard to keep up, let your care team know.

Neuropsychological testing can identify your strengths and weaknesses, and your care team can work with your school to create a plan to help address these limitations. You can also talk with your teachers/professors or school counselor about changing your schedule and adjusting deadlines.

If you're facing financial challenges, consider applying for some of the many scholarships and grants available to students who are cancer survivors.

At work

Returning to work after treatment might cause you to feel worried or concerned about how you will cope. If you were able to keep working during your treatment, the transition may come easier. If you are starting a new job or will be working with people who don't know about your illness, you have no legal obligation to

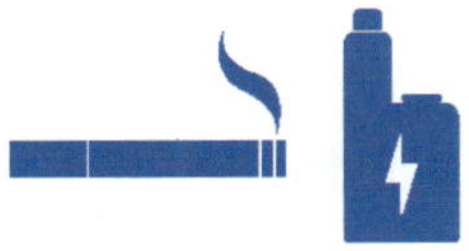

If you smoke or vape, seek help to quit

If you smoke tobacco or use e-cigarettes, it is very important to quit. Smoking can limit how well cancer treatment works. Smoking greatly increases your chances of having side effects during and after surgery. It also increases your chances of developing other cancers.

Nicotine is the chemical in tobacco that makes you want to keep smoking. Nicotine withdrawal is challenging for most smokers. The stress of having cancer may make it even harder to quit. If you smoke, ask your doctor about counseling and medicines to help you quit.

For online support, try these websites:

- SmokeFree.gov
- BeTobaccoFree.gov
- CDC.gov/tobacco

talk about your cancer history unless it directly affects your work. If you feel that letting coworkers know you are recovering from cancer treatment will be helpful, tell them. The choice is up to you.

Talk to your employer if you need to adjust things at work because of ongoing side effects. Under Federal law, employers are required to make reasonable accommodation to help you do your job during or after cancer treatment. Reasonable accommodation refers to changes that will allow you to continue to do your job without causing a significant hardship for the employer.

Recurrence

Recurrence is the return of cancer. Give yourself permission to express your feelings and reach out for help. Use your valuable time and energy to move forward. This time around you know what to expect.

- You know more. The first time, everything was a surprise. Now, you have experience.
- You have built relationships. If the same treatment team is seeing you, you are with people you already know and trust.
- You know what works for you. Instead of trial and error, you can draw on your first experience when making decisions about dealing with side effects, planning your life, and making use of support services.

Use the lessons learned during your first round of cancer to help with decision-making and take control of the situation.

> "People assume that when treatment is finished, cancer is finished. It is not that simple. The people around you return to their normal routines, but your life is forever changed. Treatment might be over, but the doctors' appointments, the side effects, the medical expenses aren't over. It wasn't until I was finished with treatment that I could even process what had happened to me. It became difficult emotionally in a whole new way."

Survivorship care plan

A survivorship care plan is a detailed plan given to you after treatment ends. It contains a summary of your treatment, along with recommendations for follow-up care. Getting follow-up care also helps check for health problems that may occur months or years after treatment ends, including other types of cancer. For AYAs, a survivorship care plan may also include information to help meet psychosocial, legal, and financial needs.

A survivorship plan should spell out who you will be seeing to monitor your health, when you should be seeing them, and what they should be doing.

Your survivorship plan should include:

- A good relationship with your primary care provider for routine health issues
- A summary of your cancer treatment history so any new doctors have a complete understanding of your case

Your survivorship plan should also include recommendations for follow-up care:

- Names and contact information for follow-up doctors
- A schedule for follow-up visits with an oncology specialist
- Routine check-ups with your primary care physician (PCP)
- Dental exam and cleaning every 6 months
- Signs and symptoms of long-term and late effects

Recommended vaccinations:

- Annual flu (influenza) vaccination
- COVID-19 vaccine and boosters
- HPV vaccination for those 9 to 26 years of age

Resources on challenges like:

- Late effects
- Anxiety, depression, and emotional distress
- Financial concerns
- Health care coverage/insurance
- Disability benefits
- Lifestyle changes (smoking cessation, nutrition, exercise)

Discuss your personalized survivorship care plan with your care team. It will contain a summary of possible long-term effects of treatment called late effects and list follow-up tests. Find out how your PCP will coordinate with specialists for your follow-up care.

More information on survivorship can be found at NCCN.org/patientguidelines and on the NCCN Patient Guides for Cancer app.

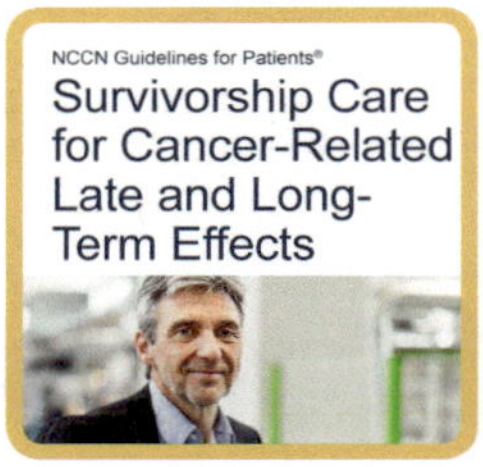

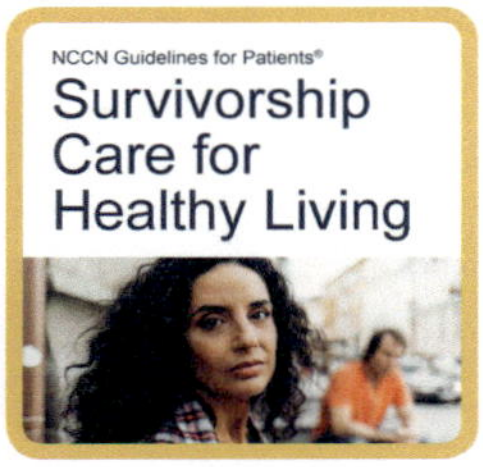

Key points

- A person is considered a cancer survivor from the time of diagnosis and throughout life.
- After treatment, you will be monitored for any new or ongoing health issues.
- AYA cancer survivors have a high risk of developing a wide range of late effects. Your risk for late effects will depend on the type(s) and length of cancer treatment you had.
- Continue to see your primary care physician (PCP) on a regular basis and have preventive cancer screenings as recommended by your PCP.
- Maintain your weight, eat a mostly plant-based diet, exercise, limit alcohol, and if you smoke or vape, seek help to quit.
- A survivorship plan should spell out who you will be seeing to monitor your health, when you should be seeing them, and what they should be doing.

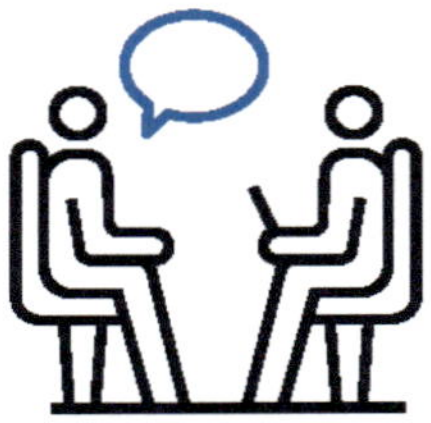

Survivorship Care Plan Examples

American Cancer Society (ACS)
cancer.org/treatment/survivorship-during-and-after-treatment/long-term-health-concerns/survivorship-care-plans.html

American Society of Clinical Oncology (ASCO)
cancer.net/survivorship/follow-care-after-cancer-treatment/asco-cancer-treatment-and-survivorship-care-plans

Centers for Disease Control and Prevention (CDC)
cdc.gov/cancer/survivors/life-after-cancer/survivorship-care-plans.htm

National Cancer Institute (NCI)
cancer.gov/about-cancer/coping/survivorship/follow-up-care

5
Care planning

This chapter provides an overview of advance care planning, survivorship care plans, palliative care, and end-of-life care.

Even when cancers are highly curable, discussion about future scenarios, including advance directives and end-of-life preferences, should begin when starting treatment. This exploration of what is important to you is often called advance care planning.

Advance care planning

Advance care planning (ACP) is making decisions now about the care you would want to receive if you become unable to speak for yourself. Advance care planning is for everyone, not just for those who are very sick. It is a way to ensure your wishes are understood and respected.

Advance care planning starts with a discussion with your care team and/or your family. Ask about your cancer prognosis and what to expect if your cancer progresses. Help your care team understand what matters to you and how you might consider "quality" of life. Discuss the medicines or therapies that best enable you to experience that quality of life. Include family, friends, and caregivers in your advance care planning. Make your wishes clear. It is important that everyone understands what you want.

You don't have to know the exact details of your prognosis. Just having a general idea will help with planning. With this information, you can decide if there is a point where you might want to stop cancer treatment. You can also decide what treatments you would want for symptom relief, such as radiation therapy, surgery, or medicine. Most people change their minds as they learn and experience more during their cancer treatment. You can change your advance care plan at any time. It is helpful to have this talk with your care team and/or friends, family, and caregivers more than once during your treatment. What you want today might change tomorrow. Making your wishes clear will ensure everyone knows what you want.

Some decisions are important to put in writing. These are called advance directives and are only a part of the larger advance care planning conversations. Advance directives include decisions about who makes decisions for you if you are too sick or unable to tell the doctors yourself, as well as the limits of what you would be willing to experience. Once you have decided, you will fill out a legal document called an advance directive that shares these details. Doctors are required by law to follow the care instructions in an advance directive. Health care professionals will not do anything that is illegal even if it is in your advance directive. This is why it is important to speak with your care team. Just like advance care plans, advance directives can change if you want them to. Frequent conversations with your care team can help.

If your family disagrees with your plan, speak to your care team. Sometimes they or other specialists can help you and your family navigate these difficult conversations. When AYAs share their wishes, families usually follow their requests, even when they would not have made the same choices themselves.

- An advance directive will include information on how much you want your doctors to do if your heart or lungs stop working or if you are no longer able to eat.
- An advance directive may ask what you would want if you had a severe disability, or were no longer able to think or act for yourself.
- Many advance directives include plans to limit what can be done if you want a natural death. Do Not Attempt Resuscitation or Do Not Resuscitate (DNAR or DNR) and Do Not Intubate (DNI) orders tell medical providers not to revive you with CPR (cardiopulmonary resuscitation) or use a breathing machine.

Name the person who will make health care decisions for you (health care proxy) in the advance directive. This person may have to make some very tough decisions. Choose carefully when selecting your proxy and make sure the proxy feels comfortable representing you.

Tell your care team and family about your advance directive and its contents. Give a copy of your advance directive to all of your doctors. Make sure the person you have chosen to speak on your behalf has a copy. Make your wishes clear. If you and your family disagree about treatment, the advance directive should reflect your wishes—not what you think your parents or partner would want. An advance directive can be changed. If your thoughts on feeding tubes or respirators change, you can change your advance directive. When you make changes, give everyone a copy of the new advance directive.

Palliative care

Palliative care is an important part of comprehensive cancer care. The goal of palliative care is to control symptoms, relieve emotional and physical suffering that comes from the diagnosis and treatment of cancer, and improve quality of life for patients and their families, regardless of the stage of the disease or the need for other therapies. Palliative care specialists are highly trained in navigating difficult conversations with patients and families, and can help you think about things like advance care planning and what is important to you. Palliative care services for AYAs are provided by a team with expertise in understanding the psychosocial, emotional, developmental, and financial issues that are unique to this age group. Sometimes, palliative care, supportive care, and best supportive care are used interchangeably.

End-of-life care

End-of-life (EOL) care provides supportive, emotional, and spiritual support. It may be called comfort care or hospice. Note that hospice is a special kind of EOL care. It refers specifically to an insurance benefit that supports those at the EOL by providing additional care providers and resources such as homecare. It also provides support to caregivers and family members. EOL discussions will include the things you have discussed in your advance care plans and advance directives, as well as your views about medical technologies and services like tube feeding and sedation, the place of death, and how to support family members and caregivers. Medically intense care at the end-of-life is more common than you might think, and it is often not what patients would have wanted for themselves. Therefore, having this difficult conservation is important.

The goal of EOL care is to give people the best life possible with the time they have left. Specifically, it aims to:

- Control symptoms
- Ease physical and emotional suffering
- Improve quality of life

Completing an advance directive to plan for end-of-life care is important. It will help you feel in control. An advance directive is a legal document that states your wishes in writing. Discuss your options for end-of life care with your care team. Ask what life might be like as your cancer progresses. Talk things over with your friends, family, and caregivers. Many AYAs want to die at home. This is not always possible. Discuss your wishes early on and throughout your treatment.

Services can be provided in your home, a hospice facility, or in the hospital. Hospice and palliative care doctors, nurses, social workers, and chaplains are experts in helping you and your family work through the spiritual and emotional challenges of coping with death. Providing support for family members is a major part of the hospice approach to end-of-life care. Most programs offer counseling and support groups for family members, including grief support.

If you have any religious or personal beliefs about certain kinds of treatment, share them with your care team.

In addition to making plans about your EOL care, organizing your personal and financial affairs can lessen the stress on family and friends after you are gone.

- Clear up any insurance questions. Find out which EOL services your provider will cover and clarify any limitations in the coverage (such as a cap on the number of visits by a nurse or health aide). Some forms of treatment may still be covered if they are being prescribed to relieve pain or symptoms.
- Organize your financial records like bank accounts, insurance policies, and mortgage to make sure your family knows where everything is. The National Cancer Institute's book, *Coping with Advanced Cancer,* (cancer.gov/publications/patient-education/advanced-cancer) has a detailed worksheet you can use.

Think about making the arrangements for a funeral or memorial service in advance.

Key points

- Advance care planning (ACP) is making decisions now about the care you would want to receive if you become unable to speak for yourself. Advance care planning is for everyone.
- An advance directive is a legal document of your wishes for treatment should you become unable to speak for yourself.
- When AYAs share their wishes, families usually follow their requests, even when they would not have made the same choices themselves.
- End-of-life (EOL) care provides supportive, emotional, and spiritual support.
- Providing support for family members is a major part of the hospice approach to EOL care.

“

Be your own advocate. Talk to someone who has gone through the same thing as you. Ask a lot of questions, even the ones you are afraid to ask. You have to protect yourself and ensure you make the best decisions for you, and get the best care for your particular situation.”

6
Making treatment decisions

It's important to be comfortable with the cancer treatment you choose. This choice starts with having an open and honest conversation with your care team.

It's your choice

In shared decision-making, you and your doctors share information, discuss the options, and agree on a treatment plan. It starts with an open and honest conversation between you and your care team.

Treatment decisions are very personal. What is important to you may not be important to someone else.

Some things that may play a role in your decision-making:

- What you want and how that might differ from what others want
- Your religious and spiritual beliefs
- Your feelings about certain treatments
- Your feelings about pain or side effects
- Cost of treatment, travel to treatment centers, and time away from school or work
- Quality of life and length of life
- How active you are and the activities that are important to you

Think about what you want from treatment. Discuss openly the risks and benefits of specific treatments and procedures. Weigh options and share concerns with your care team. If you take the time to build a relationship with your care team, it will help you feel supported when considering options and making treatment decisions.

Second opinion

It is normal to want to start treatment as soon as possible. While cancer can't be ignored, there is time to have another doctor review your test results and suggest a treatment plan. This is called getting a second opinion, and it's a normal part of cancer care. Even doctors get second opinions!

Things you can do to prepare:

- Check with your insurance company about its rules on second opinions. There may be out-of-pocket costs to see doctors who are not part of your insurance plan.
- Make plans to have copies of all your records sent to the doctor you will see for your second opinion.

Support groups

Many people diagnosed with cancer find support groups to be helpful. Support groups often include people at different stages of treatment. Some people may be newly diagnosed, while others may be finished with treatment. If your hospital or community doesn't have support groups for people with cancer, check out the websites listed in this book.

Questions to ask

Possible questions to ask your care team are listed on the following pages. Feel free to use some of these questions or come up with your own. Be clear about your goals for treatment and find out what to expect from treatment.

Questions to ask about fertility

1. Will the treatment affect my ability to have children?
2. Are there other ways to treat this cancer that will not affect my fertility?
3. How will I know if there are changes in my fertility from treatment?
4. What will be done to protect my fertility during treatment?
5. Where can I find support for coping with fertility changes?
6. After treatment ends, how long will it take for my periods to begin again?
7. If I am not having periods, should I still use contraception?
8. Is pregnancy safe for me after treatment? If so, how long should I wait after treatment to become pregnant?

Questions to ask about fertility preservation

1. Is there anything I can do after treatment to preserve my fertility?
2. What are my fertility preservation options?
3. Will any of the options affect my cancer treatment?
4. Which options will delay cancer treatment? If so, for how long?
5. Will fertility treatments increase the risk that the cancer may return?
6. How much will these fertility preservation options cost?
7. Which fertility preservation options are covered by insurance?
8. Can you refer me to a specialist who can help preserve my fertility?

Questions about testing and diagnosis

1. What type and subtype of cancer do I have? Are there any particular biomarkers or mutations present? What does this mean in terms of my prognosis and treatment options?
2. What tests do I need? What other tests do you recommend?
3. How soon will I know the results and who will explain them to me?
4. Where will the tests take place? How long will the tests take?
5. Is there a cancer center or hospital nearby that specializes in AYAs with my type and subtype cancer?
6. How do I prepare for testing?
7. Would you give me a copy of the pathology report and other test results?
8. Who will talk with me about the next steps? When?
9. Will I start treatment before the test results are in?
10. Will I have a biopsy? What type? What will be done to make me comfortable?

Questions about your care team's experience

1. What is your experience treating my type of cancer?
2. What is the experience of those on your team?
3. Do you only treat this type of cancer? What else do you treat?
4. I would like a second opinion. Is there someone you can recommend? Who can help me gather all of my records for a second opinion?
5. How many patients like me (of the same age, gender, race) have you treated?
6. Will you be consulting with experts to discuss my care? Whom will you consult?
7. How many procedures like the one you're suggesting have you done?
8. Is this treatment a major part of your practice?
9. How often is a complication expected? What are the complications?
10. Who will manage my day-to-day care?

Questions about options

1. What will happen if I do nothing?
2. How do my age, overall health, and other factors affect my options?
3. What if I am pregnant? What if I'm planning to get pregnant in the near future?
4. Am I a candidate for a clinical trial? Can I join a clinical trial at any time?
5. Which option is proven to work best for my cancer, age, and other risk factors?
6. What are the possible complications and side effects?
7. Does any option offer a long-term cancer control? Are the chances any better for one option than another? Less time-consuming? Less expensive?
8. What decisions must be made today? How long do I have to decide about treatment?
9. Is there a social worker or someone who can help me decide?
10. Is there a hospital or treatment center you can recommend for treatment? Can I go to one hospital for radiation therapy and a different center for systemic therapy?

Questions about treatment

1. What are my treatment choices? What are the benefits and risks? Which treatment do you recommend and why?
2. Does the order of treatment matter?
3. Will I have to go to the hospital or elsewhere for treatment? How often? How long is each visit? Will I have to stay overnight in the hospital or make travel plans?
4. Do I have a choice of when to begin treatment? Can I choose the days and times of treatment? Should I bring someone with me?
5. Can I stop treatment at any time? What will happen if I stop treatment?
6. How much will this treatment cost me? How much will my insurance pay for this treatment? Are there any programs to help me pay for treatment?
7. Will I miss work or school? Will I be able to drive? When will I be able to return to my normal activities?
8. What can be done to prevent or relieve the side effects of this treatment?
9. Are there any life-threatening side effects of this treatment? How will I be monitored?
10. What are the chances my cancer will return after this treatment? How will it be treated if it returns?

Questions about radiation therapy

1. What type of radiation therapy (RT) will I have?
2. What will you target?
3. What is the goal of this RT? What are the side effects?
4. How many treatment sessions will I require? Can you do a shorter course of RT?
5. Do you offer this type of RT here? If not, can you refer me to someone who does?
6. What side effects can I expect from RT?
7. Should I eat or drink before RT?
8. Will I be given medicine to help me relax during RT?
9. What should I wear?

Questions about surgery

1. What will be removed during surgery? What will this mean in terms of my recovery?
2. What kind of surgery will I have? Will I have more than one surgery?
3. Does my cancer involve any veins or arteries? How might this affect surgery?
4. How long will it take me to recover from surgery? When will I be able to return to work?
5. How much pain will I be in? What will be done to manage my pain?
6. What is the chance that this surgery will shorten my life?
7. What other side effects can I expect from surgery? What complications can occur from this surgery?
8. What treatment will I have before, during, or after surgery? What does this treatment do?

Questions about clinical trials

1. What clinical trials are available for my type of cancer?
2. What are the treatments used in the clinical trial? What does the treatment do?
3. Has the treatment been used before?
4. What are the risks and benefits of this treatment?
5. What side effects should I expect? How will the side effects be controlled?
6. How long will I be in the clinical trial?
7. Will I be able to get other treatments if this doesn't work?
8. How will you know the treatment is working?
9. Will the clinical trial cost me anything? If so, how much?
10. How do I find out about clinical trials that I can participate in? Are there online sources that I can search?

Questions about survivorship

1. What happens after treatment?
2. What are the chances that my cancer will come back or that I will get another type of cancer?
3. Who do I see for follow-up care? How often?
4. What tests will I have to monitor my health?
5. What late effects are caused by this treatment? How will these be screened?
6. What do I do if I have trouble with work or school?
7. I am looking for a survivor support group. What support groups or other resources can you recommend?

Questions about end-of-life care

1. What can I expect as my cancer progresses? How will I feel? What symptoms will I have? Will I be able to think clearly and get out of bed?
2. How much pain will I have? What can I do to ease the pain? What will you do to ease the pain?
3. How can I find out if hospice is covered by my insurance?
4. When does hospice care start? Where will my hospice care take place?
5. Does this hospital have an end-of-life support program for people my age? Please refer me to a counselor or support group who can help me and my family.

Resources

American Association for Cancer Research (AACR)
aacr.org

American Cancer Society (ACS)
cancer.org

American Society of Clinical Oncology (ASCO) For Young Adults and Teenagers
cancer.net

Be The Match®
bethematch.org

Blood & Marrow Transplant Information Network (BMT InfoNet)
bmtinfonet.org

Cancer*Care* (also available en español)
cancercare.org

Cancer Support Community
cancersupportcommunity.org/living-cancer

CaringBridge
caringbridge.org

Center for Disease Control and Prevention (CDC) (also available en español)
cdc.gov/vaccines

Chemocare
chemocare.com

Elephants and Tea
elephantsandtea.com

First Descents
firstdescents.org/programs

HPV Cancers Alliance
hpvalliance.org

MedlinePlus (also available en español)
medlineplus.gov

My Survival Story
mysurvivalstory.org

National Alliance for Mental Illness (NAMI)
nami.org

National Bone Marrow Transplant Link
nbmtlink.org

National Cancer Institute (NCI)
cancer.gov/types/aya

National Coalition for Cancer Survivorship (NCCS)
canceradvocacy.org/toolbox

National Financial Resource Directory - Patient Advocate Foundation (PAF)
patientadvocate.org/explore-our-resources/national-financial-resource-directory/

National Hospice and Palliative Care Organization (NHPCO)
caringinfo.org

National Institutes of Health (NIH)
edi.nih.gov/people

OncoLink (also available en español)
oncolink.org

Patient Access Network Foundation
panfoundation.org

Radiological Society of North America
radiologyinfo.org

Society for Adolescent Health and Medicine (SAHM)
adolescenthealth.org/Resources/Resources-for-Adolescents-and-Parents

Stupid Cancer
stupidcancer.org

Testing.com
testing.com

The Leukemia & Lymphoma Society
lls.org/PatientSupport

The Samfund
thesamfund.org

Young Adult Cancer Connection (YACC)
yacancerconnection.org

Young Survival Coalition (YSC)
youngsurvival.org

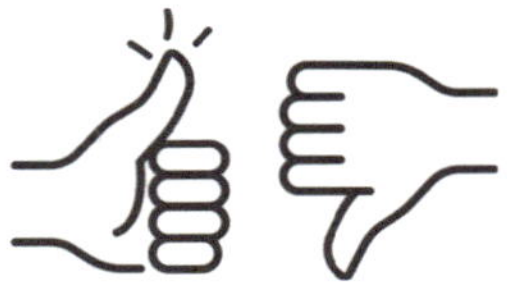

Let us know what you think!

Please take a moment to complete an online survey about the NCCN Guidelines for Patients.

NCCN.org/patients/response

Words to know

adolescents and young adults (AYA)
People who are 15 to 39 years of age.

biomarker testing
A lab test of any molecule in your body that can be measured to assess your health. Also called molecular testing.

biopsy
A procedure that removes fluid or tissue samples to be tested for a disease.

chromosome
The structures within cells that contain coded instructions for cell behavior.

clinical trial
A type of research that assesses health tests or treatments.

ejaculate
A mix of sperm and fluids. Also called semen.

fertility
The ability to produce children.

fertility preservation
A way to preserve or protect the ability to become pregnant and have a baby.

gene
Coded instructions in cells for making new cells and controlling how cells behave.

genetic mutation
An abnormal change in the coded instructions within cells.

gynecologic oncologist
A doctor who's an expert in reproductive cancers of those assigned female at birth.

hormone
A chemical in the body that triggers a response from cells or organs.

inherited mutation
A mutation passed on from parent to a child that is present before birth.

in vitro fertilization (IVF)
Procedure that removes eggs from the ovaries and combines them with sperm for fertilization in a lab.

medical oncologist
A doctor who treats cancer in adults using systemic therapy.

menopause
The end of menstrual periods.

mutation
An abnormal change in the instructions within cells for making and controlling cells.

oncofertility
Cancer doctors and reproductive experts who work together to help people keep their ability to have babies.

oncologist
A doctor who's an expert in the treatment of cancer.

oocyte preservation
The process of freezing one or more unfertilized eggs (eggs that have not been combined with sperm) to save them for future use. The eggs are thawed and fertilized in the laboratory to make embryos that can be placed in the uterus. Also called egg banking, egg cryopreservation, and egg freezing.

ovarian suppression
Methods used to lower hormone levels made by the ovaries.

ovary
One of a pair of glands that produce eggs and hormones. There is one *ovary* on each side of the uterus.

pathologist
A doctor who's an expert in testing cells and tissue to find disease.

prognosis
The pattern and outcome of a disease.

psychosocial
Having to do with the mental, emotional, social, and spiritual aspects.

psychosocial support
Support given to help meet the mental, emotional, social, and spiritual needs. Types of psychosocial support include counseling, education, group support, and spiritual support.

radiation oncologist
A doctor who's an expert in treating cancer with radiation.

radiation therapy
A treatment that uses high-energy radiation from x-rays, gamma rays, neutrons, protons, and other sources to kill cancer cells and shrink tumors.

recurrence
The return of cancer after a cancer-free period.

refractory cancer
A cancer that does not improve with treatment.

relapse
The return or worsening of cancer after a period of improvement.

reproductive system
The group of organs that work together to make a baby. They include the vagina, cervix, uterus, fallopian tubes, ovaries, penis, testicles, and prostate.

semen
The fluid that is released through the penis during orgasm. Semen is made up of sperm from the testicles and fluid from the prostate and other sex glands. Also called ejaculate.

side effect
An unhealthy or unpleasant physical or emotional response to treatment.

sperm
Cell formed in the testicle.

sperm aspiration
A procedure in which a sample of sperm cells is removed from the testicle through a small needle attached to a syringe.

sperm banking
The process of freezing sperm and storing it for future use. Samples of semen are collected and checked under a microscope in the laboratory to count sperm cells and find out how healthy they are. The sperm cells are then frozen and store. Also called sperm cryopreservation.

sperm count
A count of the number of sperm in a sample of semen. A sperm count may be used as a measure of fertility.

stem cell transplant (SCT)
A cancer treatment that replaces abnormal blood stem cells with healthy cells. Also called hematopoietic cell transplant (HCT) or bone marrow transplant (BMT).

supportive care
Treatment for the symptoms or health conditions caused by cancer or cancer treatment. Also, sometimes called palliative care or best supportive care.

systemic therapy
Cancer treatment using drugs that work throughout the body. Chemotherapy, targeted therapy, and immunotherapy are types of systemic therapy.

testicle
One of a pair of glands found inside the sac (scrotum) that produce sperm. Also called testis.

urologist
A doctor who has special training in diagnosing and treating diseases of the urinary organs in all sexes and reproductive organs in those assigned male at birth.

uterus
The organ in which a fetus (baby) grows until birth. Also called womb.

We want your feedback!

Our goal is to provide helpful and easy-to-understand information on cancer.

Take our survey to let us know what we got right and what we could do better.

NCCN.org/patients/feedback

NCCN Contributors

This patient guide is based on the NCCN Clinical Practice Guidelines in Oncology (NCCN Guidelines®) for Adolescent and Young Adult (AYA) Oncology Version 1.2023. It was adapted, reviewed, and published with help from the following people:

Dorothy A. Shead, MS
Senior Director
Patient Information Operations

Tanya Fischer, MEd, MSLIS
Senior Medical Writer

Susan Kidney
Senior Graphic Design Specialist

The NCCN Clinical Practice Guidelines in Oncology (NCCN Guidelines®) for Adolescent and Young Adult (AYA) Oncology Version 1.2023 were developed by the following NCCN Panel Members:

Smita Bhatia, MD, MPH/Chair
O'Neal Comprehensive Cancer Center at UAB

*Alberto S. Pappo, MD/Vice Chair
St. Jude Children's Research Hospital/ The University of Tennessee Health Science Center

Melissa Acquazzino, MD
Fred & Pamela Buffett Cancer Center

Wendy A. Allen-Rhoades, MD, PhD
Mayo Clinic Cancer Center

*Marie Barnett, PhD
Memorial Sloan Kettering Cancer Center

Scott C. Borinstein, MD, PhD
Vanderbilt-Ingram Cancer Center

Sun Choo, MD
UC San Diego Moores Cancer Center

Rashmi Chugh, MD
University of Michigan Rogel Cancer Center

Carrye R. Cost, MD
University of Colorado Cancer Center

Shira Dinner, MD
Robert H. Lurie Comprehensive Cancer Center of Northwestern University

*Douglas Fair, MD, MS
Huntsman Cancer Institute at the University of Utah

Noah Federman, MD
UCLA Jonsson Comprehensive Cancer Center

Jeanelle Folbrecht, PhD
City of Hope National Medical Center

Shipra Gandhi, MD
Roswell Park Comprehensive Cancer Center

*Julie Germann, PhD
UT Southwestern Simmons Comprehensive Cancer Center

Robert Goldsby, MD
UCSF Helen Diller Family Comprehensive Cancer Center

Robert Hayashi, MD
Siteman Cancer Center at Barnes-Jewish Hospital and Washington University School of Medicine

Alex Y. Huang, MD, PhD
Case Comprehensive Cancer Center/ University Hospitals Seidman Cancer Center and Cleveland Clinic Taussig Cancer Institute/University Hospitals Rainbow Babies and Children's Hospital

Mary S. Huang, MD
Dana-Farber/Brigham and Women's Cancer Center | Massachusetts General Hospital Cancer Center

*Linda A. Jacobs, PhD, CRNP
Abramson Cancer Center at the University of Pennsylvania

Cathy Lee-Miller, MD
University of Wisconsin Carbone Cancer Center

Michael P. Link, MD
Stanford Cancer Institute

John A. Livingston, MD, MS
The University of Texas MD Anderson Cancer Center

Marcio Malogolowkin, MD
UC Davis Comprehensive Cancer Center

Kevin C. Oeffinger, MD
Duke Cancer Institute

Christine A. Pratilas, MD
The Sidney Kimmel Comprehensive Cancer Center at Johns Hopkins

Damon Reed, MD
Moffitt Cancer Center

*Abby R. Rosenberg, MD, MA, MS
Fred Hutchinson Cancer Center

Tara Sanft, MD
Yale Cancer Center/Smilow Cancer Hospital

Margaret von Mehren, MD
Fox Chase Cancer Center

Nicholas Yeager, MD
The Ohio State University Comprehensive Cancer Center - James Cancer Hospital and Solove Research Institute

NCCN

Lisa Hang, PhD
Oncology Scientist/Medical Writer

Megan Lyons, MS
Guidelines Layout Specialist

* Reviewed this patient guide. For disclosures, visit NCCN.org/disclosures.

NCCN Cancer Centers

Abramson Cancer Center
at the University of Pennsylvania
Philadelphia, Pennsylvania
800.789.7366 • pennmedicine.org/cancer

Case Comprehensive Cancer Center/
University Hospitals Seidman Cancer
Center and Cleveland Clinic Taussig
Cancer Institute
Cleveland, Ohio
800.641.2422 • UH Seidman Cancer Center
uhhospitals.org/services/cancer-services
866.223.8100 • CC Taussig Cancer Institute
my.clevelandclinic.org/departments/cancer
216.844.8797 • Case CCC
case.edu/cancer

City of Hope National Medical Center
Duarte, California
800.826.4673 • cityofhope.org

Dana-Farber/Brigham and Women's
Cancer Center | Massachusetts
General Hospital Cancer Center
Boston, Massachusetts
617.732.5500 • youhaveus.org
617.726.5130
massgeneral.org/cancer-center

Duke Cancer Institute
Durham, North Carolina
888.275.3853 • dukecancerinstitute.org

Fox Chase Cancer Center
Philadelphia, Pennsylvania
888.369.2427 • foxchase.org

Fred & Pamela Buffett Cancer Center
Omaha, Nebraska
402.559.5600 • unmc.edu/cancercenter

Fred Hutchinson Cancer Center
Seattle, Washington
206.667.5000 • fredhutch.org

Huntsman Cancer Institute
at the University of Utah
Salt Lake City, Utah
800.824.2073 • huntsmancancer.org

Indiana University
Melvin and Bren Simon
Comprehensive Cancer Center
Indianapolis, Indiana
888.600.4822 • www.cancer.iu.edu

Mayo Clinic Cancer Center
Phoenix/Scottsdale, Arizona
Jacksonville, Florida
Rochester, Minnesota
480.301.8000 • Arizona
904.953.0853 • Florida
507.538.3270 • Minnesota
mayoclinic.org/cancercenter

Memorial Sloan Kettering
Cancer Center
New York, New York
800.525.2225 • mskcc.org

Moffitt Cancer Center
Tampa, Florida
888.663.3488 • moffitt.org

O'Neal Comprehensive
Cancer Center at UAB
Birmingham, Alabama
800.822.0933 • uab.edu/onealcancercenter

Robert H. Lurie Comprehensive Cancer
Center of Northwestern University
Chicago, Illinois
866.587.4322 • cancer.northwestern.edu

Roswell Park Comprehensive
Cancer Center
Buffalo, New York
877.275.7724 • roswellpark.org

Siteman Cancer Center at Barnes-
Jewish Hospital and Washington
University School of Medicine
St. Louis, Missouri
800.600.3606 • siteman.wustl.edu

St. Jude Children's
Research Hospital/
The University of Tennessee
Health Science Center
Memphis, Tennessee
866.278.5833 • stjude.org
901.448.5500 • uthsc.edu

Stanford Cancer Institute
Stanford, California
877.668.7535 • cancer.stanford.edu

The Ohio State University
Comprehensive Cancer Center -
James Cancer Hospital and
Solove Research Institute
Columbus, Ohio
800.293.5066 • cancer.osu.edu

The Sidney Kimmel Comprehensive
Cancer Center at Johns Hopkins
Baltimore, Maryland
410.955.8964
www.hopkinskimmelcancercenter.org

The University of Texas
MD Anderson Cancer Center
Houston, Texas
844.269.5922 • mdanderson.org

UC Davis
Comprehensive Cancer Center
Sacramento, California
916.734.5959 • 800.770.9261
health.ucdavis.edu/cancer

UC San Diego Moores Cancer Center
La Jolla, California
858.822.6100 • cancer.ucsd.edu

UCLA Jonsson
Comprehensive Cancer Center
Los Angeles, California
310.825.5268 • cancer.ucla.edu

UCSF Helen Diller Family
Comprehensive Cancer Center
San Francisco, California
800.689.8273 • cancer.ucsf.edu

University of Colorado Cancer Center
Aurora, Colorado
720.848.0300 • coloradocancercenter.org

University of Michigan
Rogel Cancer Center
Ann Arbor, Michigan
800.865.1125 • rogelcancercenter.org

University of Wisconsin
Carbone Cancer Center
Madison, Wisconsin
608.265.1700 • uwhealth.org/cancer

UT Southwestern Simmons
Comprehensive Cancer Center
Dallas, Texas
214.648.3111 • utsouthwestern.edu/simmons

Vanderbilt-Ingram Cancer Center
Nashville, Tennessee
877.936.8422 • vicc.org

Yale Cancer Center/
Smilow Cancer Hospital
New Haven, Connecticut
855.4.SMILOW • yalecancercenter.org

Notes

Index

Made in the USA
Monee, IL
05 November 2026

67379964R00040